Caregiver Therapy

Caregiver Therapy

written by
Julie Kuebelbeck and
Victoria O'Connor

illustrated by
R.W. Alley

ONE
CARING
PLACE

Abbey Press

Text © 1995 Julie Kuebelbeck and Victoria O'Connor
Illustrations © 1995 St. Meinrad Archabbey
Published by One Caring Place
Abbey Press
St. Meinrad, Indiana 47577

Library of Congress Catalog Number
95-77810

ISBN 0-87029-285-4

Printed in the United States of America

Foreword

Caregiving can be a rewarding and life-affirming experience. It can also be draining and exhausting. Whether you give care to others as a professional, a volunteer, a relative, or a friend, you can sometimes forget about your own needs. Yet to effectively take care of others you must take care of yourself.

Caregiver Therapy can help you keep your life in balance as you care for others—an achievement that takes dedication and conscious living. Its guidelines invite you to be faithful to your needs and boundaries, to replenish yourself, to seek support, to pray. As you learn to treat yourself with compassion and love, you become more able to do the same for others.

Caregiver Therapy also suggests ways to deepen and enrich your caregiving experience—as you open your heart to others during difficult times, as you open your spirit to lessons of love and trust. These pages will remind you that handling yourself and others with care truly does make a difference in the world.

1.

Living fully includes caring for yourself and giving care to others. Keeping both in balance will make your journey through life rich and rewarding.

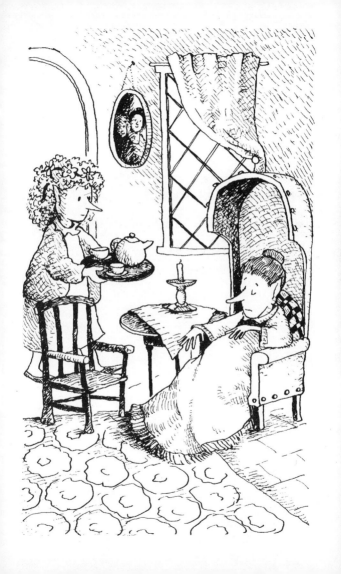

2.

Giving care is sacred.
Recognize that your actions
are prayer in motion.

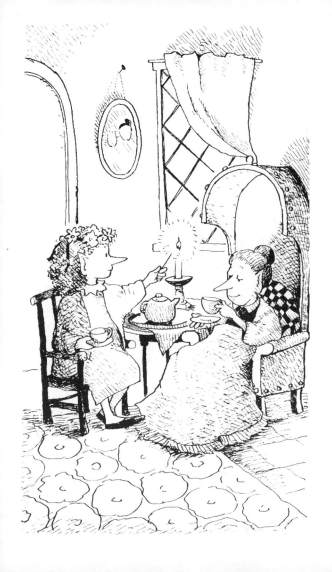

3.

Value the gifts of caregiving.
It's an opportunity to grow in
tolerance, patience, compassion,
and understanding of the
limitless power of love.

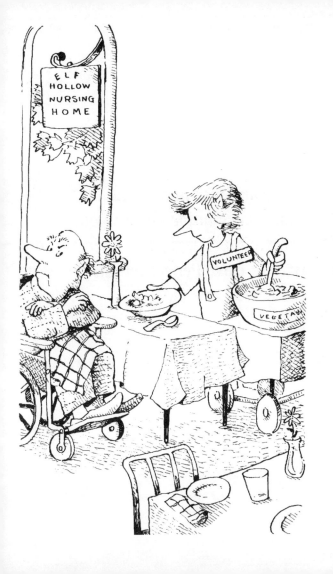

4.

Let your wise and gentle inner voice guide you in your caregiving. There's no "perfect" way to care. Perfection isn't the goal. Love is.

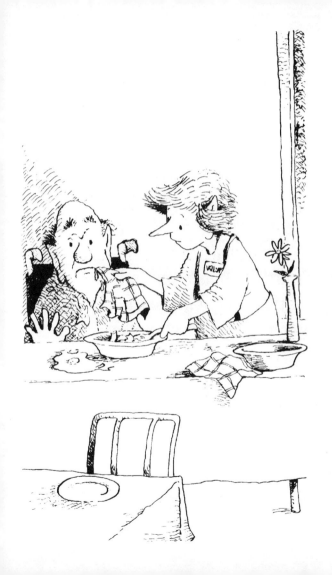

5.

Sometimes helping others means allowing them to give. A homemade card, a smile, a heartfelt "thank you" are gifts to be treasured. Graciously accept what others have to offer.

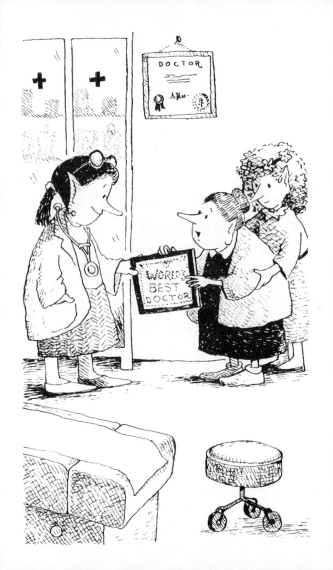

6.

You needn't guess at what is helpful to others. Ask what would be of most benefit to them right now. Their needs may change from moment to moment, from day to day. Remain flexible and open.

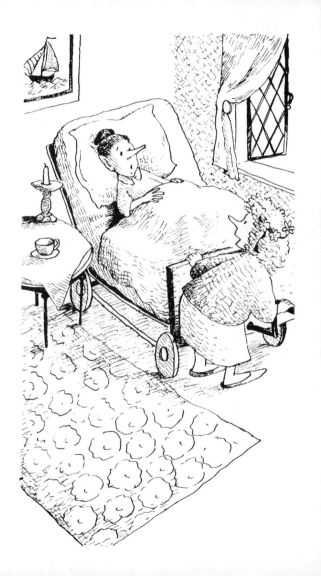

7.

Prayer can bring comfort
to those in need. When
appropriate, ask, "Would
you like me to pray with you?"
You can also pray privately for
someone in your care. Have
faith and pray simply.

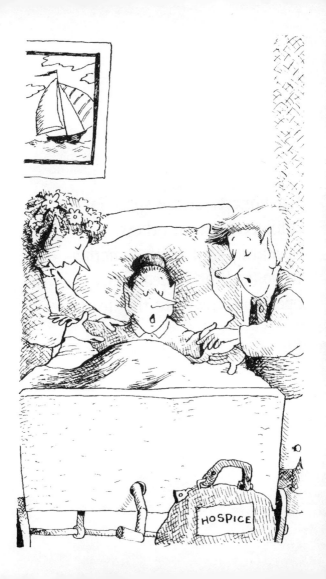

8.

Let honesty create space for connecting with others. Speaking your truth, whether to yourself or someone else, opens pathways to the heart.

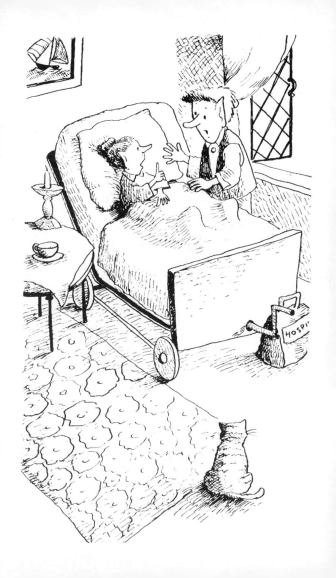

9.

One of the greatest expressions
of love is to meet people exactly
where they are. Allow others to
learn their life lessons the way
they need to. Trust God to guide
them through their process.

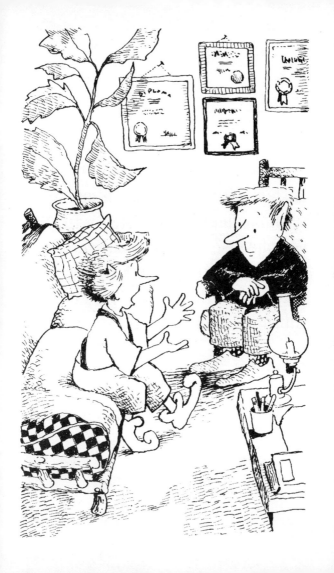

10.

Listen with full attention and without judgment. Listen with your heart as well as your ears. Soulful listening is a powerful way to let others know they are valued and cared about.

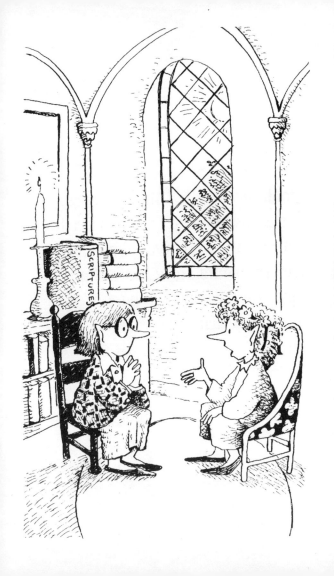

11.

People need to tell their stories as a way to come to terms with changes in their lives. You may hear the same story more than once. Be patient. It's part of emotional healing.

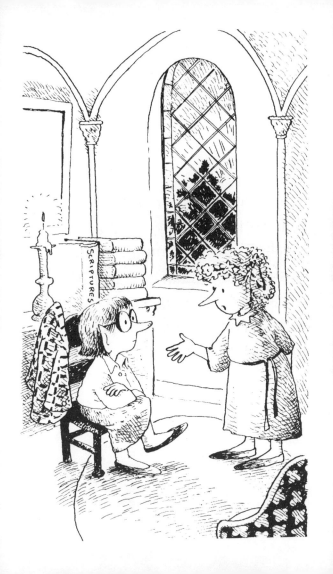

12.

Soothe and comfort with well-timed and appropriate touch. Your hand on an arm or shoulder, a hug, or a gentle massage for a homebound patient can provide support, connection, and healing.

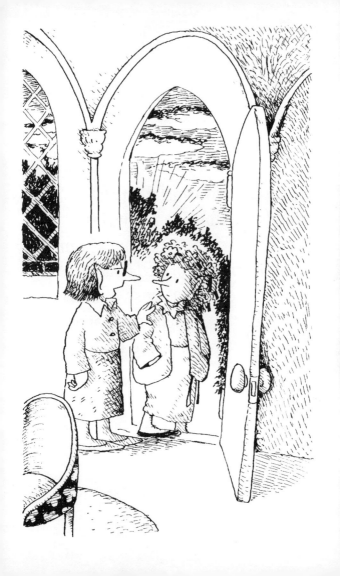

13.

Be aware of miracles in the mundane. Routine activities and chores may sometimes seem unexciting and of little value, but an energizing sense of order and accomplishment can come from taking care of the basics.

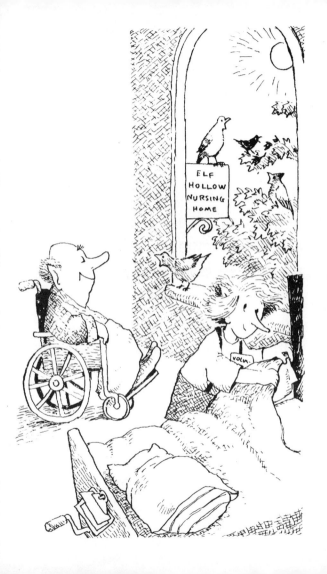

14.

Be spontaneous. Smile. Laugh hard. Sing songs. Tell jokes. Celebrate birthdays. Fill the room with signs of joy and life! Everyone gives and receives much in an atmosphere of lightness.

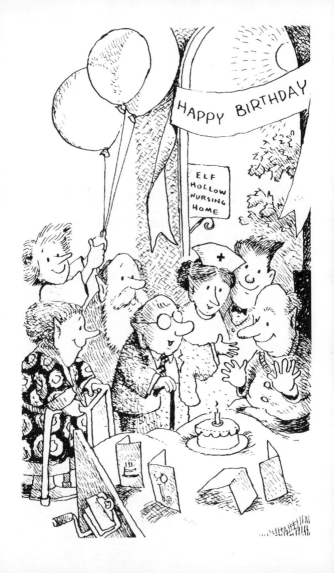

15.

Self-care is an essential part of caregiving. If you feel guilty when you want to take time off and care for yourself, remember you can give more freely and effectively when you've replenished yourself.

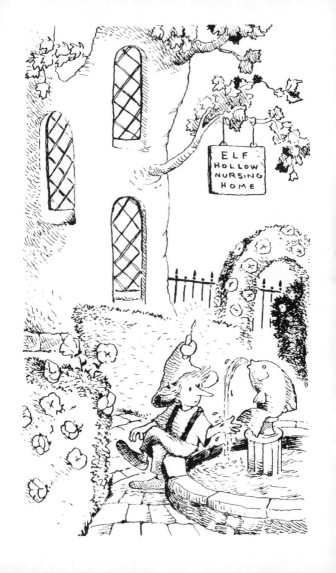

16.

Respect your own needs and boundaries. Others feel freer to ask for what they want if they know you'll take care of yourself and say no when you must. And you'll better understand the needs of others when you meet your own needs.

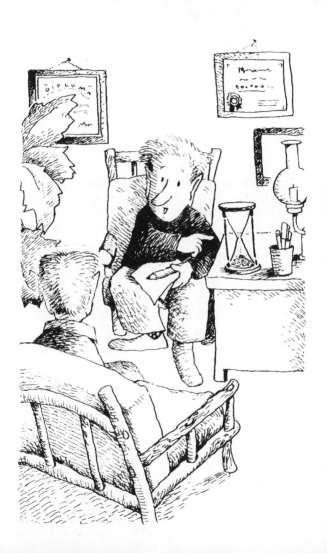

17.

The responsibility of caring for another can be physically, mentally, and emotionally overwhelming. Have a support network—of friends or other caregivers—who will listen, understand, and ease your burden.

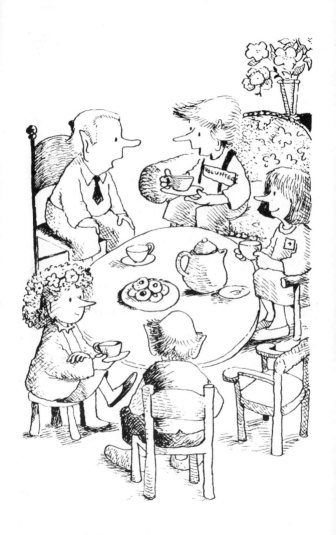

18.

When you feel depleted and
empty, remember life's energy
is always there to support you.
Taking a nap, watching
sunlight play in the trees, or
listening to inspiring music
will help remind your body,
mind, and spirit that there
is strength to go on.

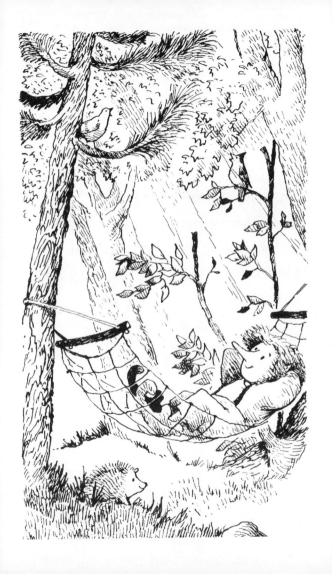

19.

Lovingly honor your body's needs. Movement and exercise can revitalize every part of you; wholesome foods and rest will nourish you.

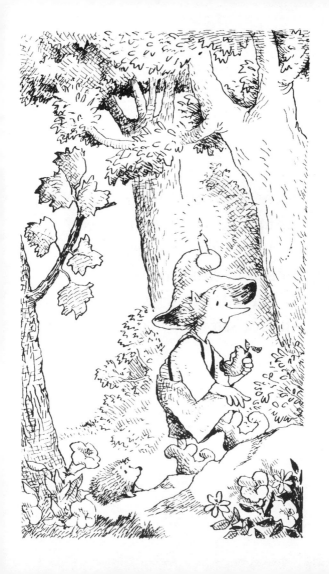

20.

Renew your mind with meditation. Know that all is well while you take a few minutes to clear your head and reconnect with your intuitive self.

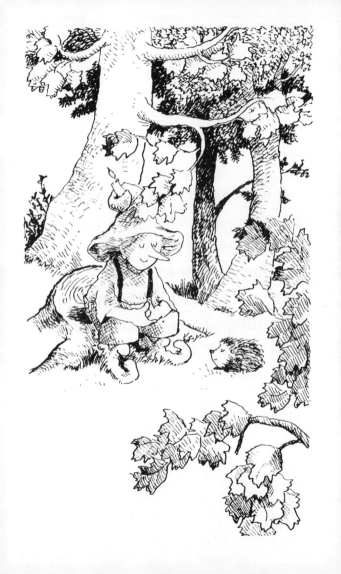

21.

If you're caring for a loved one at home, you need respite from your caregiving role. Provide time for yourself and give others an opportunity to help by turning to your friends, relatives, church, and community.

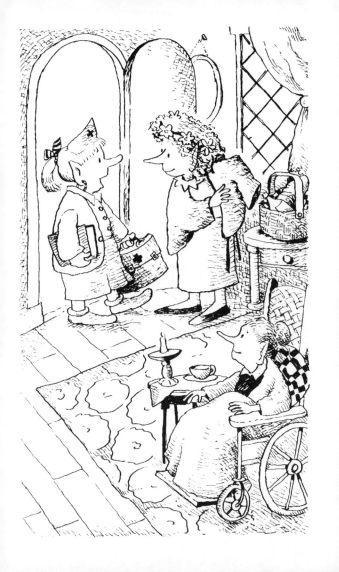

22.

An occasional escape from
everyday reality can restore
your vitality. Go to the movies,
watch your favorite sitcom,
share a chocolate sundae with
a friend.

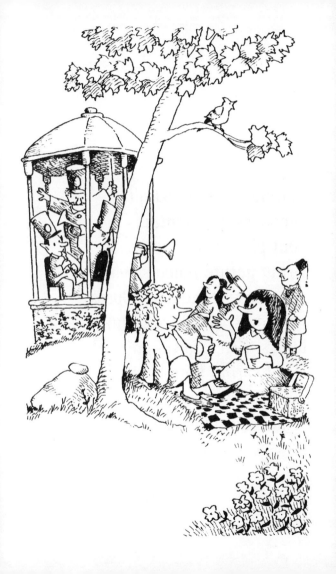

23.

Nature soothes, delights, energizes, and reminds you of your place in the universe. Bring nature indoors when you can't be outside. Open windows, gather autumn leaves, listen to the rain, smell spring flowers, make circles of stones. Enjoy the solace nature brings.

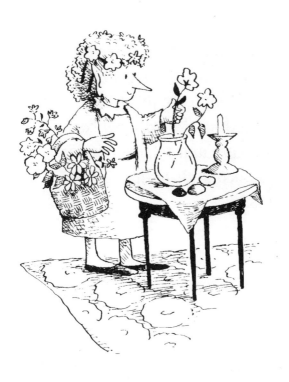

24.

Be mindful of the centering power of breath for yourself and the one you care for. Following the rhythm of breathing can calm fears and relieve tension for someone in pain or under stress.

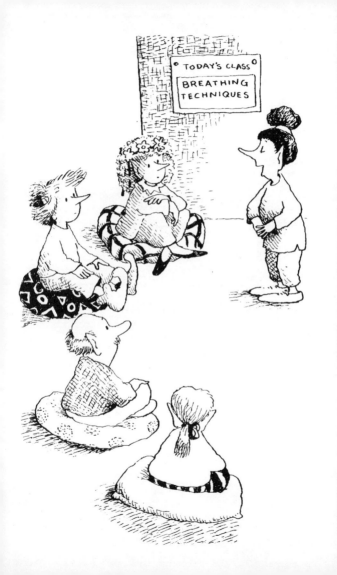

25.

Record your experiences, feelings, frustrations, and desires in a special book. Your journal will become your memory, your truth, and your friend.

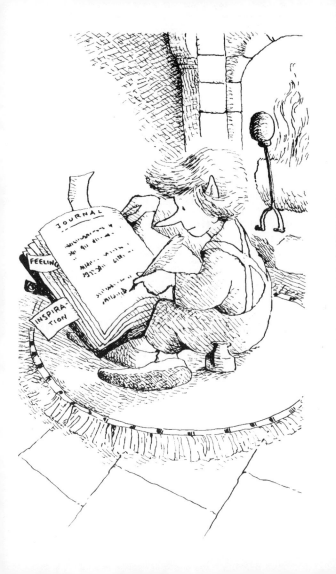

26.

If you're feeling desperate to help, take a moment to see if you're wanting to rescue, change, or manage some person or situation. Others' lives are not yours to control. Learn to lovingly detach and trust their process.

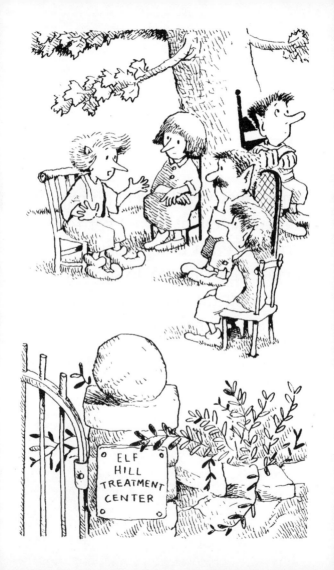

27.

Sometimes when you're giving care, others may choose not to receive. When this happens, honor their right to do so, and know that the time will come to offer your help again.

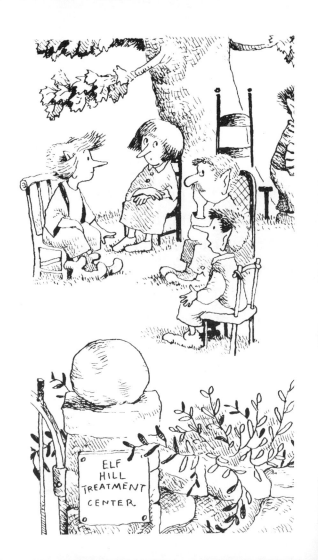

ELF
HILL
TREATMENT
CENTER.

28.

You may feel angry at times in your caregiving. Maybe there's been unclear communication or you've forgotten to take care of yourself. Find a safe and appropriate way to express your anger, and know it will clear the path for closeness and love.

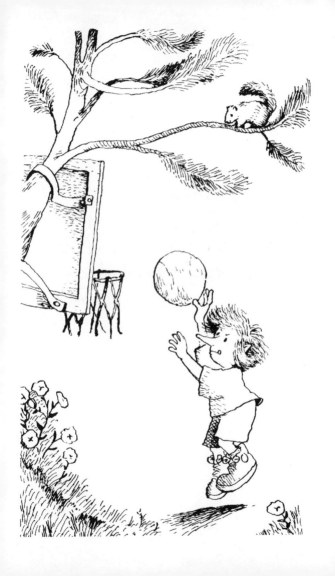

29.

Practice gratitude. It lightens your load, softens your heart, and reminds you to let go of the outcome. Being grateful paves the way for acceptance.

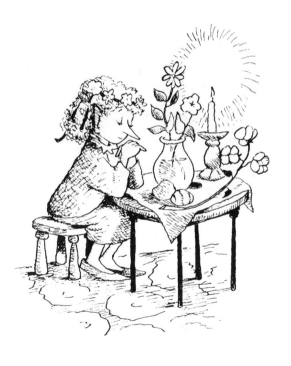

30.

Be open to the newness and
significance of each moment.
Within it lies the chance to
experience the richness of
emotion, the freedom of
spontaneity, the depth of
the human spirit.

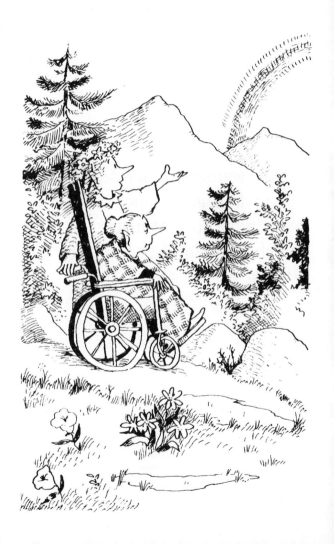

31.

Forgive yourself for not being able to do it all or make everything better. Whatever you choose to give is a unique gift and will be enough.

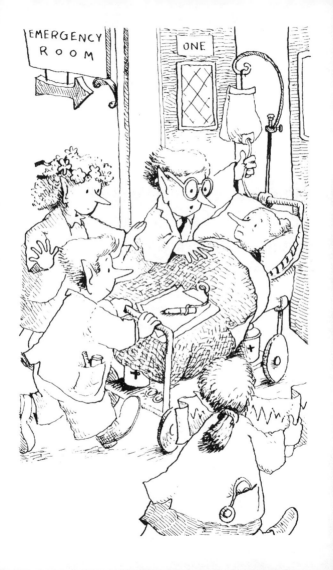

32.

When you feel alone and in need, let God care for you. God is the greatest caregiver there is.

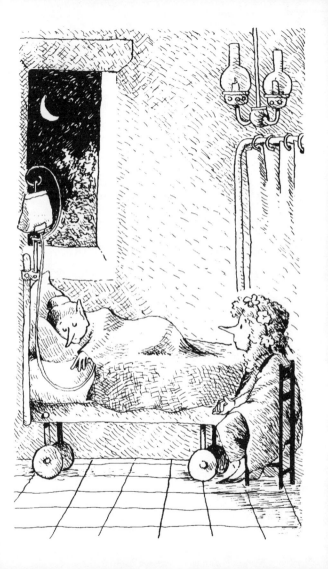

33.

When it seems there's nothing more you can do for someone, the most loving thing may be to hold that person gently in your heart.

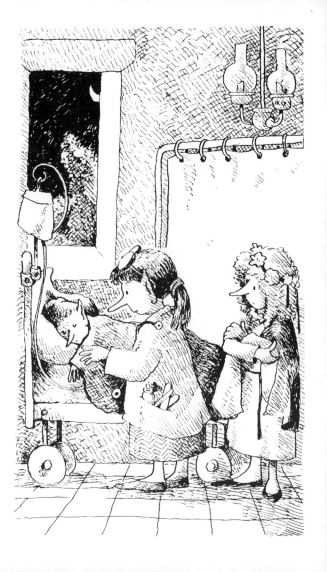

34.

The loss of someone you have cared for will bring feelings of sadness and grief. Be gentle with yourself; make time to be with your pain. Moving through your feelings will eventually provide resolution and healing.

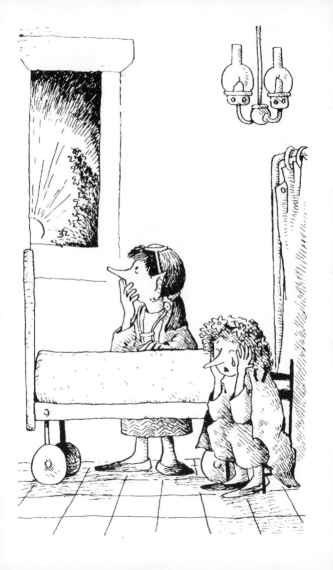

35.

Watch and welcome the sunrise. Amid confusion and uncertainty, it reminds you that darkness does turn to light and that a loving force is in charge of the universe.

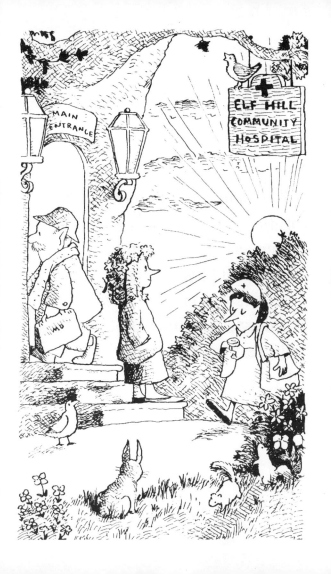

36.

When someone you have cared for dies, a sense of relief may accompany your feelings of sadness and loss. This is a common response for caregivers. Acknowledge this and other feelings that arise. They're all part of grieving.

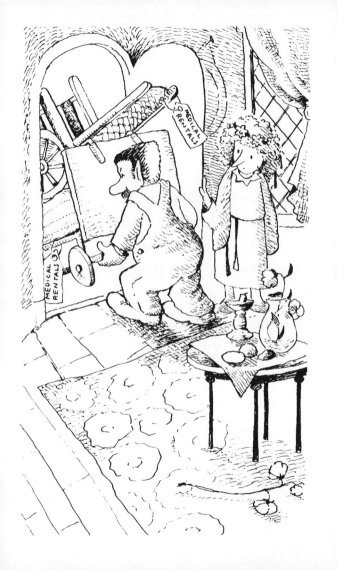

37.

Savor those moments when you see the effect of your caregiving on another's life. There will be other times when you won't know the impact you've had. Always trust that what you do is part of the bigger picture and everything is exactly as it needs to be.

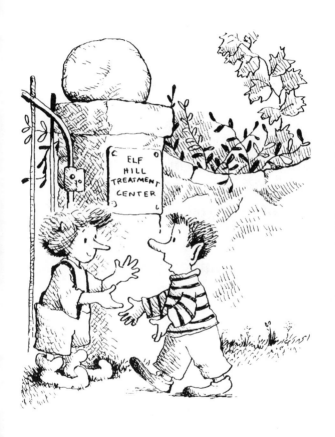

38.

Each time you choose to handle someone with care, you make a significant difference in the world. Applaud yourself for having the love, strength, and courage to care!

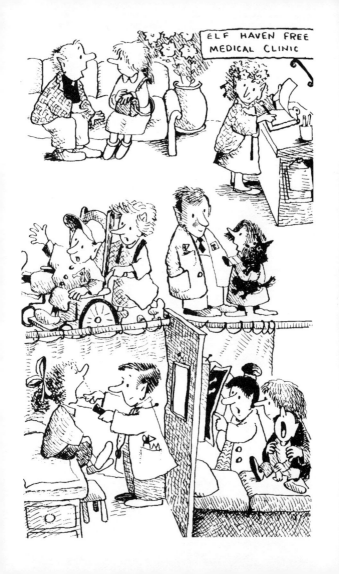

Victoria O'Connor is an artist, manager, movement therapy graduate, and co-creator of Purple Porcupine Greetings. Her recovery process and studies have taught her the significance of giving care to herself as well as to others. She lives with her husband, John, in Hastings, Minnesota.

Julie Kuebelbeck served five years as a volunteer working with bone marrow transplant patients at the Fred Hutchinson Cancer Research Center in Seattle, Washington. Since 1991, she has been a hospice volunteer, assisting patients and families as they cope with the daily task of caring for loved ones at home. She's learned through experience the importance of balance between self-care and caregiving. She resides in Seattle, where she is co-creator of Purple Porcupine Greetings, studies yoga, and enjoys the people and outdoors of the Northwest.

Illustrator for the Abbey Press Elf-help Books, **R.W. Alley** also illustrates and writes children's books. He lives in Barrington, Rhode Island, with his wife, daughter, and son.

The Story of the Abbey Press Elves

The engaging figures that populate the Abbey Press "elf-help" line of publications and products first appeared in 1987 on the pages of a small self-help book called *Be-good-to-yourself Therapy*. Shaped by the publishing staff's vision and defined in R.W. Alley's inventive illustrations, they lived out author Cherry Hartman's gentle, self-nurturing advice with charm, poignancy, and humor.

Reader response was so enthusiastic that more Elf-help Books were soon under way, a still-growing series that has inspired a line of related gift products.

The especially endearing character featured in the early books—sporting a cap with a mood-changing candle in its peak—has since been joined by a spirited female elf with flowers in her hair.

These two exuberant, sensitive, resourceful, kindhearted, lovable sprites, along with their lively elfin community, reveal what's truly important as they offer messages of joy and wonder, playfulness and co-creation, wholeness and serenity, the miracle of life and the mystery of God's love.

With wisdom and whimsy, these little creatures with long noses demonstrate the elf-help way to a rich and fulfilling life.

Elf-help Books

...adding "a little character" and a lot
of help to self-help reading!

New Baby Therapy	#20140
Grief Therapy for Men	#20141
Teacher Therapy	#20145
Stress Therapy	#20153
Making-sense-out-of-suffering Therapy	#20156
Get Well Therapy	#20157
Anger Therapy	#20127
Caregiver Therapy	#20164
Self-esteem Therapy	#20165
Take-charge-of-your-life Therapy	#20168
Everyday-courage Therapy	#20167
Peace Therapy	#20176
Friendship Therapy	#20174
Christmas Therapy (color edition) $5.95	#20175
Grief Therapy	#20178
Happy Birthday Therapy	#20181
Forgiveness Therapy	#20184
Keep-life-simple Therapy	#20185
Celebrate-your-womanhood Therapy	#20189

Acceptance Therapy (color edition) $5.95   #20182

Acceptance Therapy   #20190

Keeping-up-your-spirits Therapy   #20195

Slow-down Therapy   #20203

One-day-at-a-time Therapy   #20204

Prayer Therapy   #20206

Be-good-to-your-marriage Therapy   #20205

Be-good-to-yourself Therapy   #20196
(hardcover) $10.95

Be-good-to-yourself Therapy   #20255

Book price is $4.95 unless otherwise noted.
Available at your favorite giftshop or bookstore—
or directly from One Caring Place, Abbey Press
Publications, St. Meinrad, IN 47577.
Or call 1-800-325-2511.
www.carenotes.com